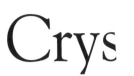

Crys...s

How to c...
for over 20 occasions

Michael Gienger

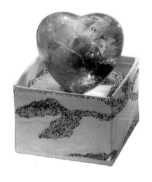

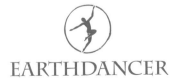

EARTHDANCER

A FINDHORN PRESS IMPRINT

First edition 2015

Crystal Gifts
Michael Gienger

This English edition © 2015 Earthdancer GmbH
English translation © 2014 JMS books LLP
Editing by JMS books LLP (www.jmseditorial.com)

Originally published in German as *Ein Stein für jeden Anlass*
World Copyright © Neue Erde GmbH 2013
All rights reserved

Title page:
Photo: Karola Sieber
Design: Dragon Design UK Ltd.

Photos: All photos by Karola Sieber, www.makrogalerie.de, with the exception of the following pages: 18–19 Aldo Murillo/iStock.com; 26–27: SelectStock/iStock.com; 34–35 MNStudio/shutterstock.com; 38–39 Carmen Martinez Bamùs/iStock.com; 42–43 Simone Becchetti/iStock.com; 58–59 stockstudioX/iStock.com; 82–83 Wesley Thornberry/iStock.com

Typesetting and design: Dragon Design UK Ltd.
Typeset in News Gothic

Printed and bound in China by Midas Printing Ltd.

ISBN 978-1-84409-665-7

Published by Earthdancer GmbH, an imprint of:
Findhorn Press, 117–121 High Street,
Forres, IV36 1AB, Scotland.
www.earthdancerbooks.com, www.findhornpress.com

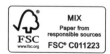

MIX
Paper from
responsible sources
FSC® C011223

Contents

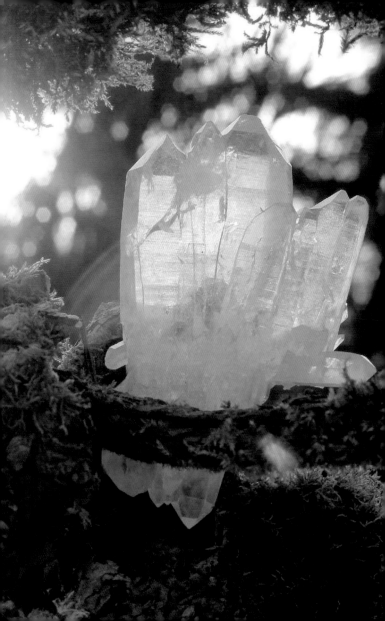

The message of crystals

Silent and yet still able to communicate, stones deliver their messages wordlessly, reaching out to us, touching our hearts to be understood by our whole being. When presented as gifts, they are a beautiful way of expressing good wishes, of offering greetings or congratulations – and they can help those wishes come true.

Crystal gifts and greetings are messages of a very special kind: crystals bring strength and joy; they help us to recuperate from illness, are a source of protection and power, and also help to promote trust and bring comfort.

Crystals express affection in their own way, preserving the memory of special moments and events through their very existence.

Stones are more than mere words. We can see, touch and feel them, we can carry them or hold them in our hands; they make good companions in both good and bad times. They are enduring gifts, patient, always there for us, ready for when we need them. It is time to give them – and us – the chance to speak...

Michael Gienger has been putting into words what crystals have to tell us for 25 years. In this book, he expresses their message with warmth, displaying a deep understanding of crystals and people, giving wonderful voice to the silent language of the stones. His carefully chosen words open us up to the gift of crystals.

Crystals simply are.
They remain and are just the way they are.
Their very being is their message.
How they became
Is a reflection of the way we too are made.

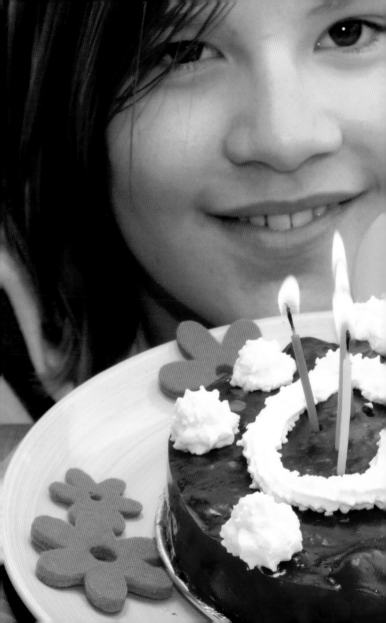

Birthdays

The anniversary of our birth comes around once again, reminding us of the different talents and traits we have been developing since the day we were born. A birthday is a day to celebrate our very existence and the gifts we bring to the world. It is the day we celebrate that we are the way we are. And in return for the fact that we give ourselves to the world, all our wishes will come true.

Crystal messages for a birthday

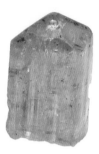

Gold topaz

I wish you every happiness on your birthday! May your sun shine, today and every day. Stay just the way you are and be yourself. You have many gifts – don't hide them, we can't wait to see what you can do.

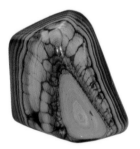

Malachite

Life is an adventure. Every day is different and every moment is new – I wish you wonderful surprises and exciting challenges in a life that is beautiful, fulfilling and intense.

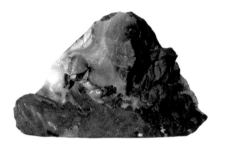

Precious opal

Life is colourful, life is beautiful – may every day be like a birthday for you. May you savour every joy, contentment and happiness, and a life full of colours that never fade. The most beautiful jewel is you!

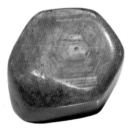

Ruby

Let your fire burn brightly. You are precious and I dearly hope that your wishes come true. Grab life with both hands and live! May the rhythm of life carry you along until you find what you truly want.

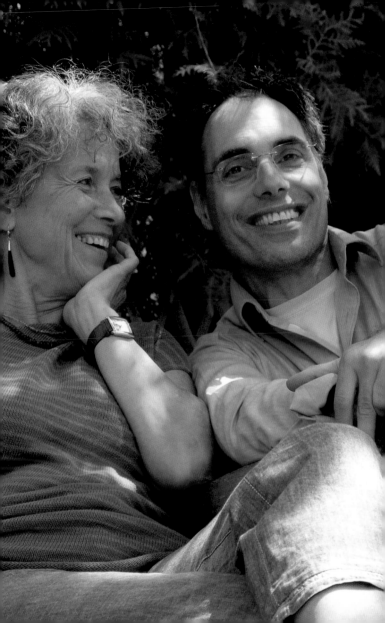

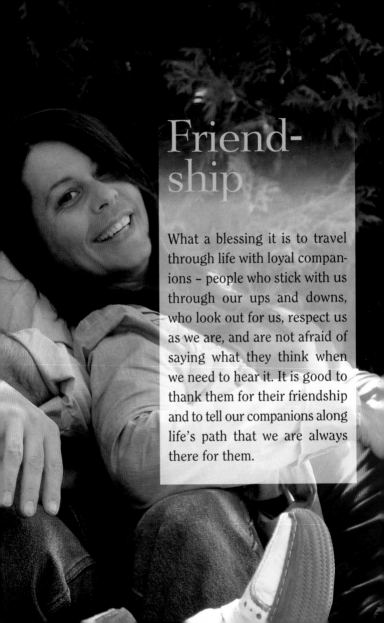

Friend-ship

What a blessing it is to travel through life with loyal companions – people who stick with us through our ups and downs, who look out for us, respect us as we are, and are not afraid of saying what they think when we need to hear it. It is good to thank them for their friendship and to tell our companions along life's path that we are always there for them.

Crystal messages for friends

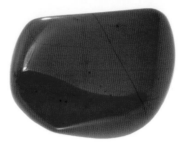

Jasper

I can rely on you. You are there when I need you and are often my rock in a stormy sea. I feel strong with you at my side and I will happily give you all my strength, too; together, we are unbeatable!

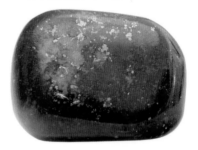

Lapis lazuli

Thank you for your friendship and understanding; for every sincere word and for allowing me to be myself with you. The time we spend together is genuine and precious and our friendship is a gift.

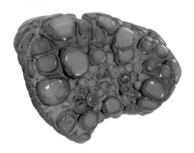

Malachite

It is good to go through thick and thin with you, conquering the world and enjoying adventures together. We both love to experience new things and solve life's puzzles – life is more intense and beautiful when we make the journey together.

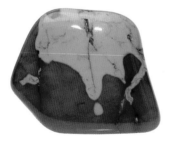

Mookaite

Life with you is a joy. How much fun we have had, how much pleasure we have found in simple things – with you life is never boring and every day is different. The world is full of colour and sunshine – it is great that you're there for me.

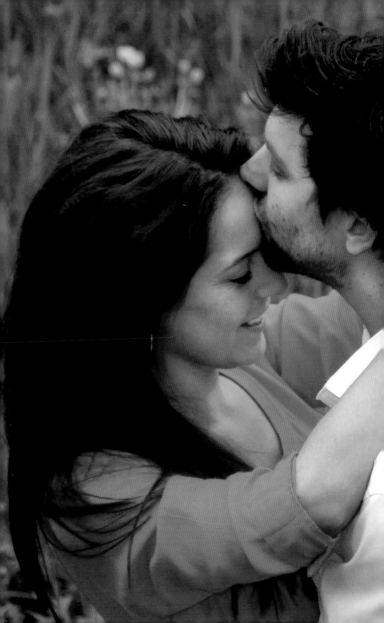

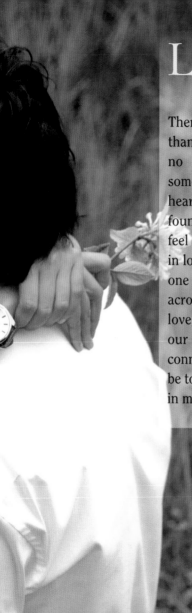

Love

There is no greater happiness than knowing we are loved, no greater joy than loving someone else. Love allows our hearts to meet, to make a profoundly deep connection, to feel an intense emotion. When in love, we are always close to one another, at any time and across any distance. When in love, we discover the root of our desire to reach out and connect with someone and to be together, finding happiness in making one another happy.

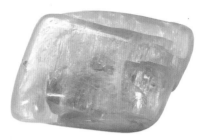

Kunzite

I love you because you are the way you are. I long for you when we are separated – and I am all the more joyful when we are together. I embrace both our being apart and together – and I embrace you, just the way you are.

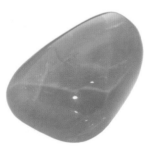

Rose quartz

My heart leaps when I see you. And it races when you are near. I feel at peace with you. Hours, days, years pass while I am wrapped up in the nearness of you. May the moment last; you, who are my life, stay close to me...

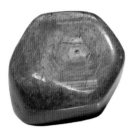

Ruby

How happy I am that we have found one another. What a joy it is that you are here. You light up my heart – when you are with me, all is well. We can conquer the world together and dance our way through life – I love you!

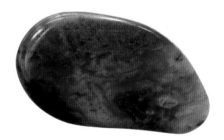

Thulite

I want to touch you tenderly, kiss you passionately and seduce you, sharing desire and joy with you – not tomorrow, today! I want to experience love, laughter and passion with you and feel you near me all day and all night.

Wedding

The decision to journey along life's path together, side by side, through the good times and the bad, comes from deep within our hearts in a moment of silence. Once shared with the world, the celebration that follows strengthens and validates these vows. But only when they are renewed and affirmed on a daily basis will they become an eternal bond or a 'marriage' – the closest connection between two people.

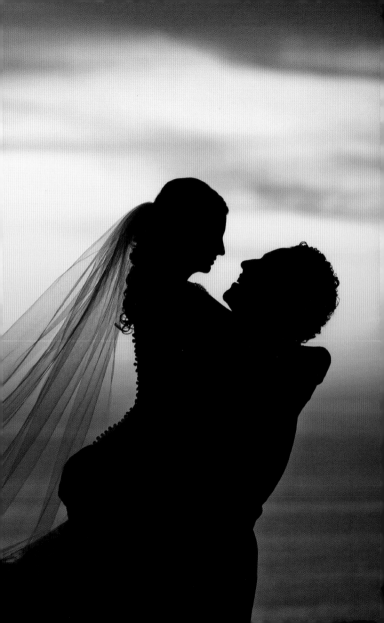

Crystal messages for weddings

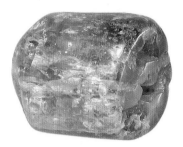

Aquamarine

Our lives should be joined as one, a shared journey of countless steps. We will follow our paths through the world together, at each other's side for as far as our minds can see in time and space.

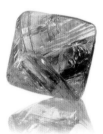

Diamond

I will always be true to you and remain steadfastly loyal at your side. My decision to go through life with you is clear and made with a pure heart. May honesty and truth now be with us in our thoughts, words and deeds.

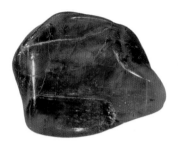

Emerald

I rejoice every day that you are by my side. I feel closer and closer to you with every day that passes. You bring harmony and beauty into my life and I am happy when our thoughts are as one. I love you!

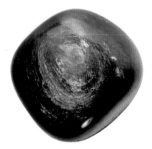

Sapphire

The only conditions or demands placed on our love will be to cherish one another just as we are. Being free together, never alone, with truth forming the basis of our marriage, may we always be bound, heart to heart, in deep understanding.

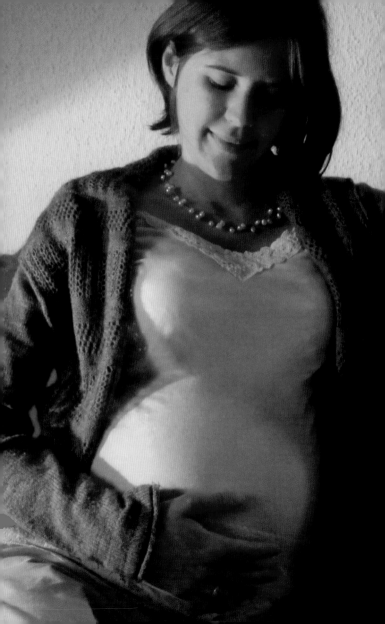

Pregnancy

An unborn child is growing, a new life has been created and one of the greatest miracles is about to take place. This new life needs care, protection, security, nourishment and vitality in order to develop and grow. The child has found its home inside the mother, who begins to prepare another home for her newborn child; both mother and child are beginning a new life together.

Crystal messages for pregnancy

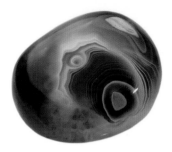

Agate

Everything will be fine. This new life will develop in safety and security. All is in place and provided for; life nourishes us all. Feel secure and strengthened, mother and child, you are both strong enough to take this great step!

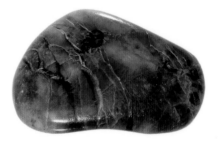

Chrysocolla

Life is the power within everything, bringing each of Nature's seeds to fruition. Life is the greatest power in Nature and it has now awoken once again. Trust the life that carries and cares for you, and feel that you're alive – every day!

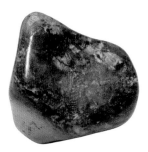

Dumortierite

Don't worry. What will this new life be like? Nobody knows or can know, but if you take it easy, it will be easy. So enjoy your time of pregnancy while you hope for the very best, and look forward to the future, whatever it may hold...

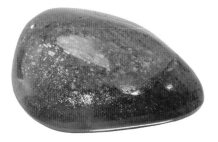

Sunstone

Child, you are a gift who brings new life. And as a mother you too are a gift, having carried that child. Together you will see life's new dawn, delivering joy and new discoveries.

Birth

The baby has arrived and begun its life on Earth, in a big, wide world full of colour and exciting discoveries. It is lovely to welcome a child – a joy for the parents of every newborn and a promise of the future. The child's path through life is yet to begin, life is still all about the here and now, and being part of that is every newborn's first gift to its parents. It is good to say thank you and to reward yourself, too.

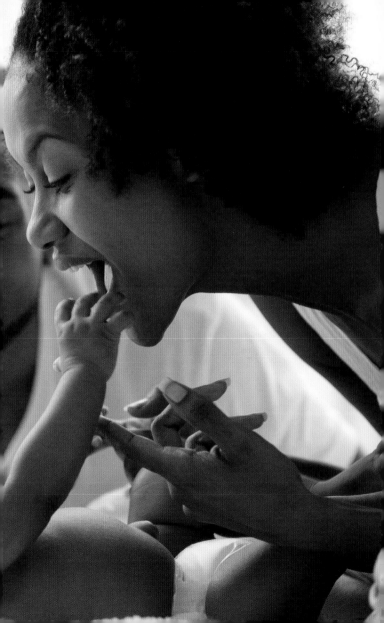

Crystal messages for newborns

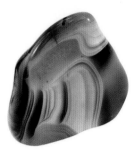

Agate
We are there for you! We are delighted you have joined us and we welcome you with open arms. Feel safe among us, cherished and protected. Come here in peace and begin your life.

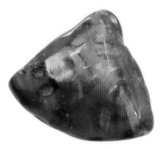

Amber
A little ray of sunshine! We wish you a life full of joy and happiness. You will soon learn to sink your teeth into life (and you will soon have small teeth for that very purpose), and we hope you enjoy every moment. Let your laughter ring out.

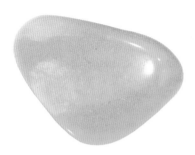

Calcite

You're getting bigger as each day passes, all by yourself; little by little and day by day, you are growing into your body. Learn to use it and see what you can do. Let your body grow and flourish, it will soon be your best friend.

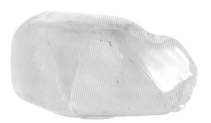

Rose quartz

It's wonderful to have you with us! You have come just to us, touching us deeply and bringing joy, so we give you our love from the bottom of our hearts, now and throughout your life.

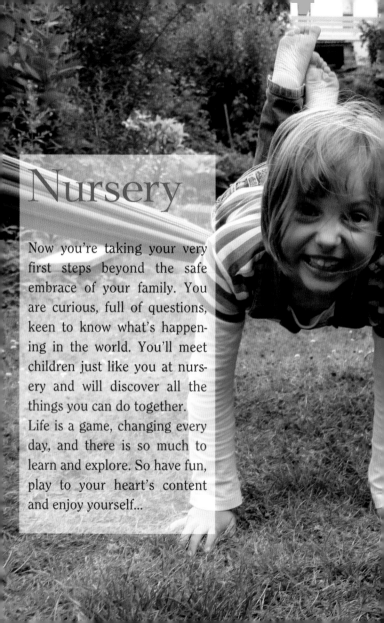

Nursery

Now you're taking your very first steps beyond the safe embrace of your family. You are curious, full of questions, keen to know what's happening in the world. You'll meet children just like you at nursery and will discover all the things you can do together.

Life is a game, changing every day, and there is so much to learn and explore. So have fun, play to your heart's content and enjoy yourself...

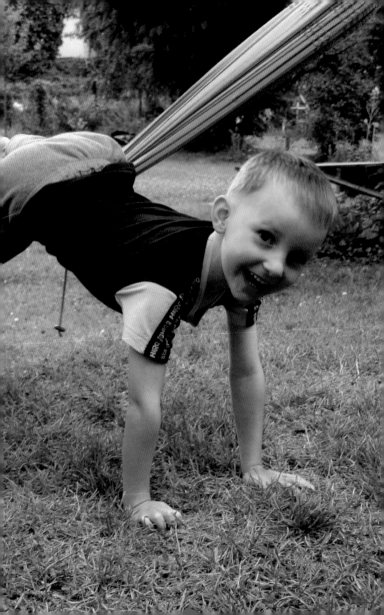

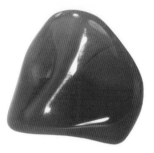

Carnelian

Your encounters with other people will be different every day: today they might be great fun, but tomorrow there might be arguments and conflict. Learn to hold your own and to understand others. Making friends is wonderful – it's easier to do things together in this world.

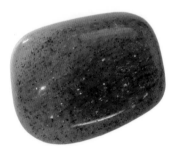

Green aventurine quartz

Just look at everything there is to explore! Life is a game, full of ideas and surprises. Try everything you can and see what others are doing. You won't always get it right first time, but don't get fed up, you'll soon get the hang of it...

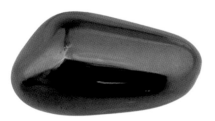

Hematite

Just feel how strong you are! You may only be small, but you are extremely determined and this will help you to overcome every difficulty; you will develop skills day by day. Learn, practise and never give up – that's the way to tackle life.

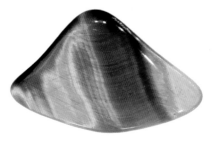

Tiger's eye

Not every idea is a good one, and you won't like everything that other people want to do. Understand that and learn to say no. Don't lose heart and look at what makes you happy – especially when life isn't going well and you are feeling sad.

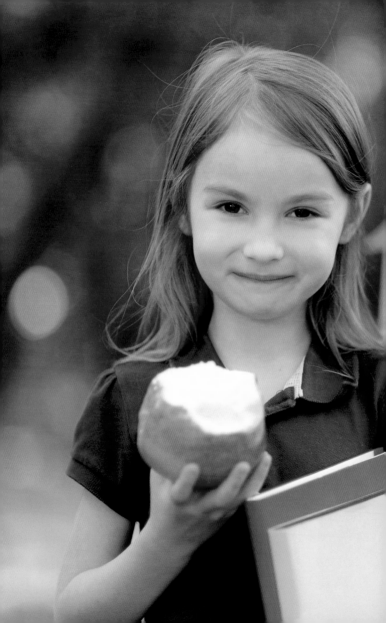

Starting school

You want to know more. You want to learn. You have great expectations of the world – will they be met? Now you're going to school, happy, excited, even a little scared? You will be taught many things, but what you learn is up to you and is your choice. You have to decide for yourself what is true or false, what is useful and good – you'll work it out, trust yourself, you can do it!

Crystal messages for starting school

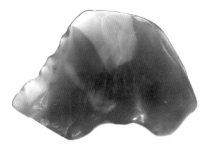

Blue chalcedony

You are smart! Keep your eyes and ears open and your studies will be easy. New experiences await you every day – make the most of them and try things out for yourself. Speak honestly and listen to what others have to say.

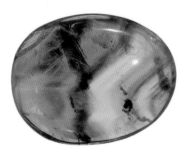

Fluorite

Studying isn't always easy, sometimes it makes you tired and your head feels too full of information. Be wary of this and anything you may have missed as a result. Do this and you will be amazed at how much you will be able to learn, retain and remember.

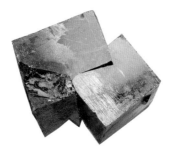

Pyrite
Never stop asking questions. The secrets of the world are there to be discovered. The things you see, hear, feel and know will remain with you throughout your life.

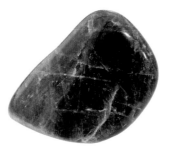

Sodalite
What your parents and teachers tell you is not necessarily always correct; they do not know and understand everything there is to know and understand in this world. Think for yourself, weigh up what you are told and discover the truth for yourself – this knowledge will stay with you forever.

Growing up

You are no longer a child, but a young person wanting to grow up and become an adult. 'Who am I?' is your most important question – you are certainly not like everyone else. Discovering what makes you different, finding companionship and friends, breaking boundaries, standing up for your rights, doing what you have to and taking on responsibility is not always easy – but it is the only way to find out what you are really made of.

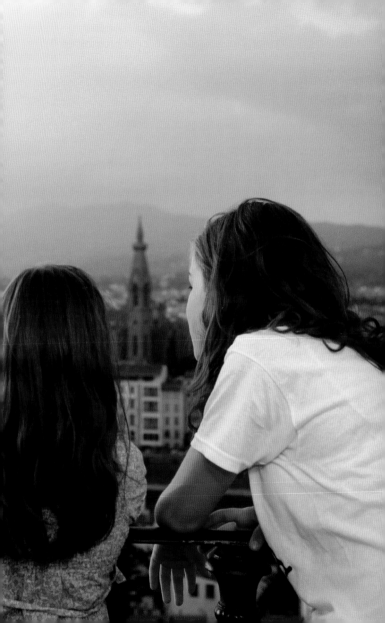

Crystals messages for children growing up

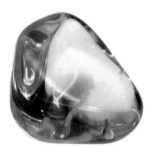

Citrine

Life should be a joy, and you have a right to be yourself. Uncertainty can only be overcome through action and experience, while self-confidence and the courage to deal with life come with success and maturity. Believe in yourself enough to put yourself to the test.

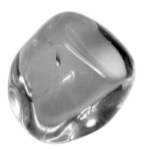

Clear quartz

Our sight is crystal clear when we see things as they really are. It is the only way we can recognise ourselves and understand the world – and the only way to change those things that require improvement. We are now responsible for our own lives...

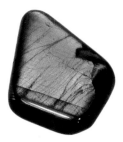

Labradorite

What is truth and what is illusion? Do you want to see behind the mirror? Don't just believe what people tell you, but try things out and judge them for yourself before you reject them. It will shatter some illusions but will also bring you insight.

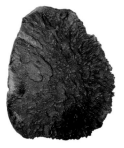

Moldavite

Freedom! Making your own decisions, instead of people making them for you – deciding for yourself what you want and what you don't want. This is your right, so make your choice. Responsibility means accepting the consequences of your actions and this marks the path to adulthood.

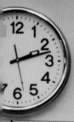

Exams

Exams play a decisive and fateful role in your life. You can prepare for them well with study, practice and coaching, but until the time comes, you cannot know exactly what the challenge will be or how you will cope with it. Exams mirror life in that sense, offering us a glimpse of ourselves; in terms of results, whatever will be, will be – simply sitting the exam is already a victory in itself!

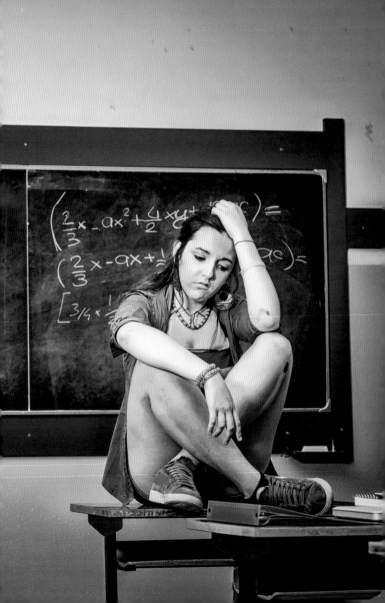

Crystal messages for taking exams

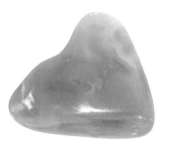

Blue chalcedony

Stay calm. Have confidence that when the time comes you will know what to do or say. When something comes to mind, be sincere. Trust in your knowledge to express yourself in the right way.

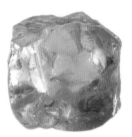

Chrysoberyl

Be prepared. Make an early start on your studies and work steadily – you can do it. It will help to avoid pressure and stress, and the ability to be disciplined and persevere will soon follow. Fear of failure will disappear and you will know what you know. You will do it!

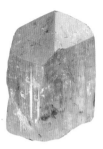

Gold topaz

You can do it. You've got it in you. Just feel your power and your strength. Your abilities give you confidence and success is assured. You will draw greater strength from the knowledge that you have done it than from the results. You did it!

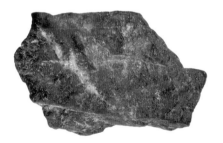

Lapis lazuli

Exam time is your own time. Be yourself, you are at your best just as you are. Think your own thoughts and do things your way, using your knowledge. Then you will be fully in charge and have the situation totally in hand.

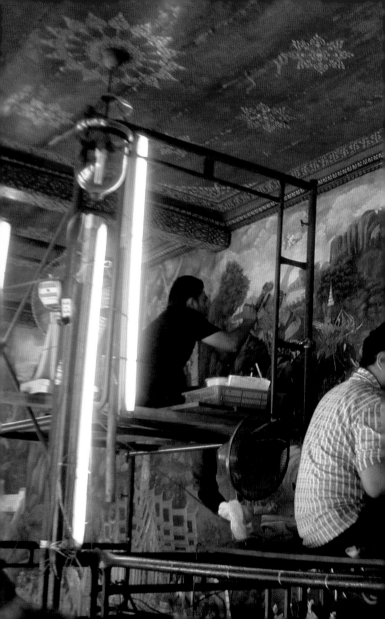

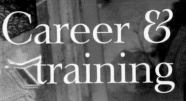

Career & training

What will be my contribution in life? What will be my career, my vocation? Choosing a career sets the course for your whole life. Should you be guided by your skills and preferences? Whether you are still making or have already made that choice, professional success and fulfilment will follow when you engage fully and make a conscious effort to give and to contribute.

Crystal messages for choosing a career

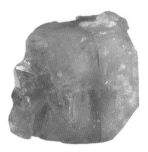

Apophyllite

Recognise both your potential and your limitations. Don't put yourself under pressure or set your sights too high – be honest with yourself. Find a career that encourages your personal development to flourish and take responsibility for your actions.

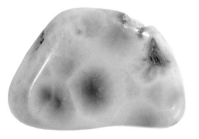

Larimar

Follow your intuition if you feel any doubts holding you back. Your life is your own and you set the boundaries. Be guided by what you want to contribute – the choice is yours, which also means that you can change your mind!

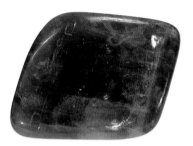

Multi-coloured tourmaline

Be guided by what you deem reasonable. See what your actions can achieve in the world, what you can contribute with your talents. Give yourself enough space to allow your different skills to develop.

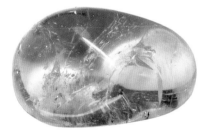

Topaz

You can achieve your goals! Anything is possible if you are prepared to commit to it heart and soul. Don't opt for what seems to be the easy option, choose what is really important to you. Be guided by your desires and abilities.

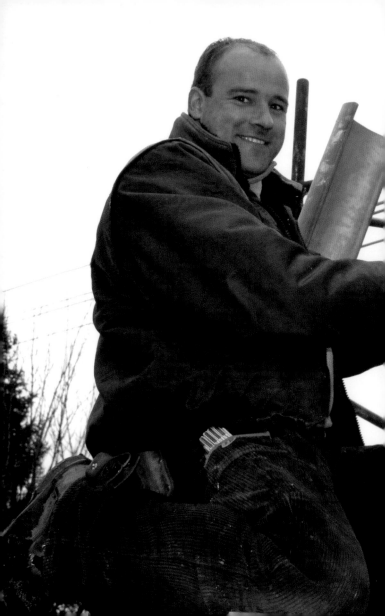

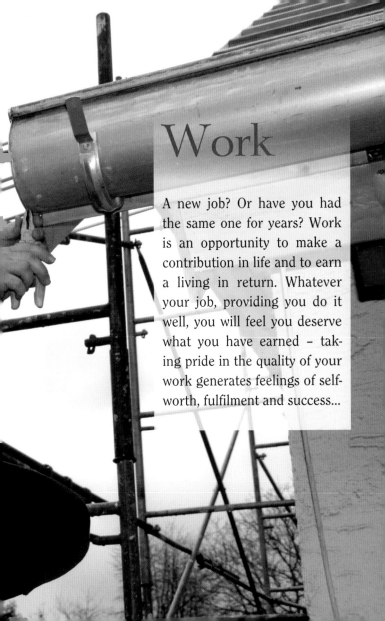

Work

A new job? Or have you had the same one for years? Work is an opportunity to make a contribution in life and to earn a living in return. Whatever your job, providing you do it well, you will feel you deserve what you have earned – taking pride in the quality of your work generates feelings of self-worth, fulfilment and success...

Crystal messages for work or a new job

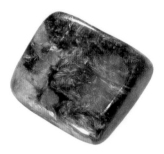

Charoite

Engage and get involved, but spend your energy wisely and you will be able to achieve a great deal. Be sure to finish what you start and your energy will be renewed. Being aware of your abilities frees you from stress and anxiety; you will succeed in whatever you undertake.

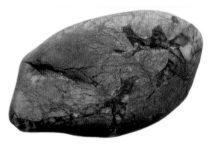

Purpurite

Give yourself some space when you are pushing yourself too hard. Remember what your goals are and keep them in mind. It will give you strength and free up your creativity. New ideas lead to new opportunities.

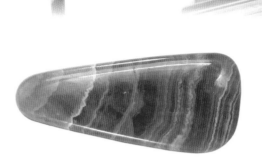

Rhodochrosite

Each day is different, even if it involves the same daily tasks. Always embrace the job at hand and respect what you have achieved. In this way you will find pleasure in your work and an ability to complete it with ease.

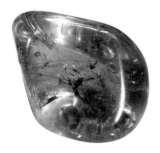

Smoky quartz

Your inner strength is always greater than the challenges you face. Being aware of this frees you from stress and helps you get to grips with things properly. Recognise the simple solutions and organise your work sensibly – success and contentment will follow.

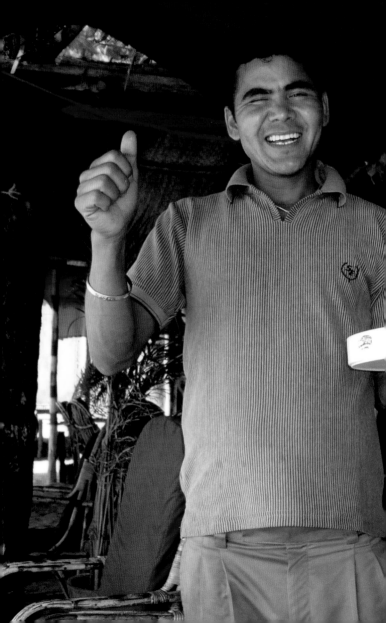

Business start-up

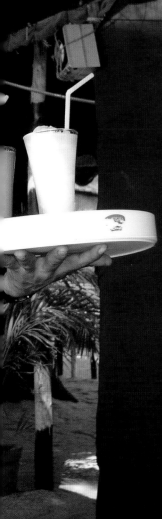

In your own business you can decide what your contribution to life will be. However, with every enterprise comes the risk of success and failure, so it is good to be aware of your capabilities and your limitations. When competent people provide support, you will benefit from their good advice. Courage, hard work and skill will all be required, not to mention a little luck.

Crystal messages for business start-ups

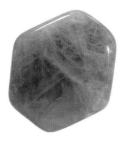

Aquamarine

Pursue your path in business with purpose and keep an eye out for every potential opportunity. Life is change, and being aware of this is the secret to success. Always keep up to date with market trends and demands.

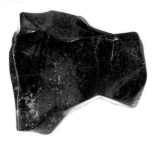

Lapis lazuli

Keep learning and be confident of your abilities. Take responsibility for your actions and use your energy wisely – this will help you avoid mistakes, limit any damage that may result and increase your chances of success.

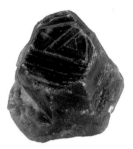

Sapphire

Be careful what you wish for, it might come true! Take time to think before you start, note what happens and check the result. The more clearly you know where you want to go, the more certain you will be of reaching that destination.

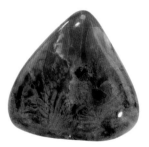

Sugilite

Never compromise your principles, even when temptation is there to cloud your judgement. Sincerity and honesty are worth much more than quick profit. It can help you forge reliable partnerships and ensure success in the long term.

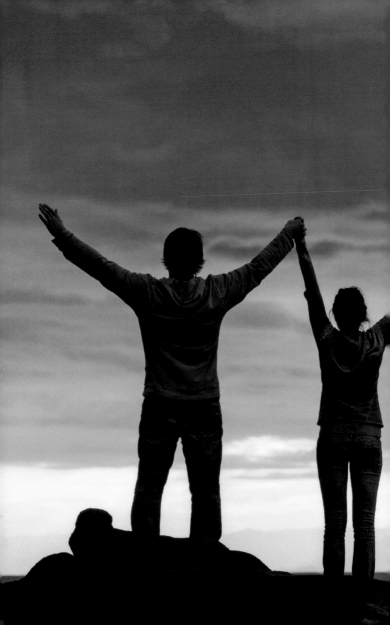

Success

When wishes come true, when hard work bears fruit, when efforts yield results and endeavours achieve their goal – that is success! It follows effort, just as the harvest follows the sewing of seeds. Behind every wish for 'the best of luck' lie both skill and determination, and if things work out, celebrate your success ...

Crystal messages for success

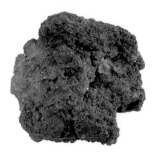

Azurite

Within every thought lie the seeds of its realisation. Recognise how you have contributed to your own success and it will not be your last idea. What you thought was 'accidental' happened because you were open and ready for it.

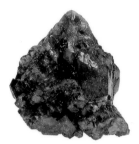

Dioptase

Everything you have achieved is yours, make the most of it! You are allowed to be rich, successful and happy. Look at those you can help with the fruits of your hard work – shared gifts multiply and you get out of life what you put in.

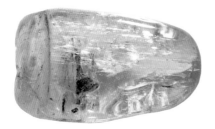

Gold topaz

Enjoy your victories and be glad – don't underplay them or hide your light under a bushel. Celebrate your success and broadcast it – and inspire others to be just as successful.

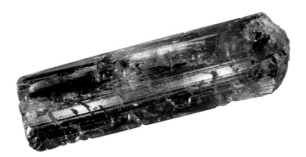

Multi-coloured tourmaline

To make many wishes come true, you have to act with resolve. Patience and perseverance, generosity and amiability, understanding and sympathy – such qualities behind success will continue to bear fruit, and their rewards will increase when you share them with others.

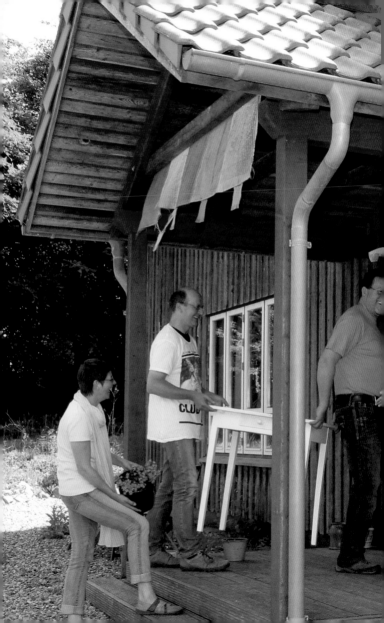

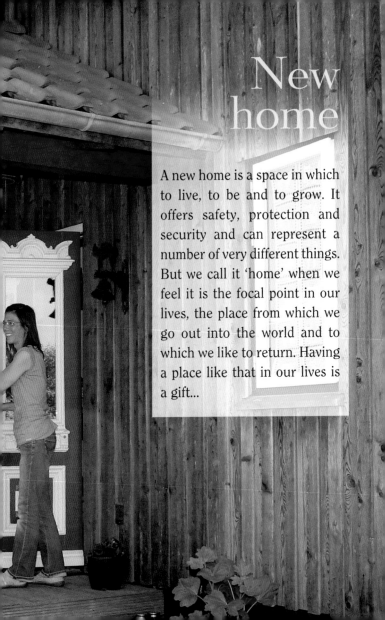

New home

A new home is a space in which to live, to be and to grow. It offers safety, protection and security and can represent a number of very different things. But we call it 'home' when we feel it is the focal point in our lives, the place from which we go out into the world and to which we like to return. Having a place like that in our lives is a gift...

Crystal messages for a new home

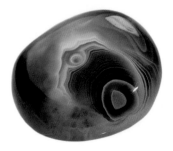

Agate

May your new house truly be a home – a place that nourishes and protects you, a place that you carry within you, even when you are far away. May you always be welcomed with security and warmth when you enter its doors.

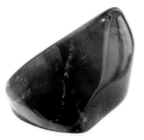

Amethyst

May peace always reign in your home and may you be free of all burdens when you are inside it. Just as it is easier to breathe freely in fresh air, may the atmosphere around you remain pure and may your life be free, easy and long...

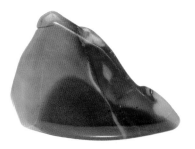

Mookaite

May there always be life within your four walls, along with companionship, joy and a welcome for friends. May all those who come to visit bring gifts, all those who stay a while feel at ease, and all those who enter leave feeling stronger.

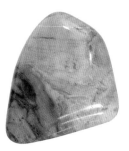

Petrified wood

May your home be a place where you can put down roots like a tree in fertile soil. May it give you strength, allowing you to grow and many others to draw support from its strong trunk, finding food and shelter beneath its spreading branches.

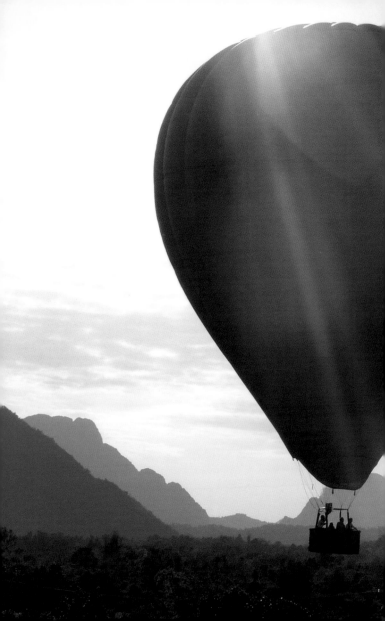

Travel

What is a good journey? One that sees you reach your destination safely, without being too dull? One full of adventure but not danger? Journeys seldom turn out as planned, and therein lies their charm. They remove us from our everyday world and offer new experiences. So we wish you 'bon voyage!' on journeys that exceed all expectations, take you to your destination unharmed and and provide some good stories along the way...

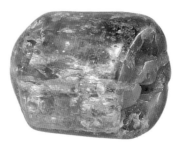

Aquamarine

Even the longest journey starts with a single step. Make sure that you keep your goal in mind – but keep your eyes open for every detail and opportunity you encounter on the way. Travelling with this kind of attitude makes the journey the destination...

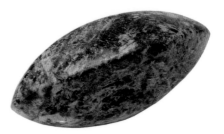

Dumortierite

May you complete your journey with ease and cheerfulness and without difficulty, going wherever you wish. Anxiety and concern should ease until they trouble you no longer and your journey will be stimulating and interesting.

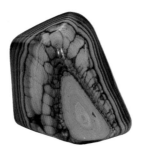

Malachite

You know what you are hoping for, but you don't know what to expect. Every journey is full of surprises. Seek out and embrace the unexpected. Don't shy away from adventure and you will be richly rewarded.

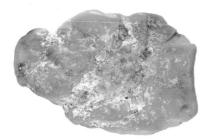

Turquoise

May you avoid all danger and arrive safely at your destination. May good fortune guide you along the right paths, even when these may sometimes appear long and winding. May you always be granted a safe return.

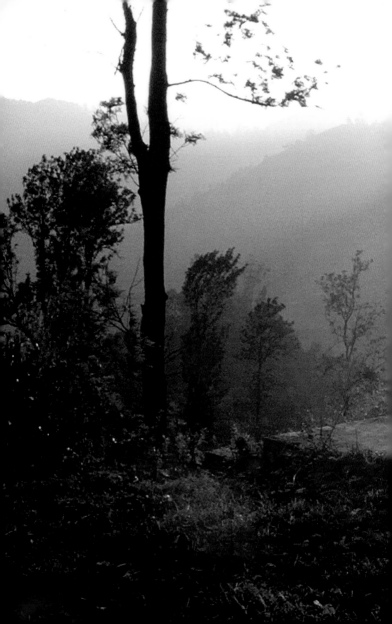

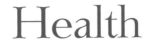

Health

Good health is something that we often learn to appreciate when it is taken from us. It is only when we are sick that we truly value what we used to take for granted. When wishing that someone gets well soon and returns to good health, we should also hope that they will recognise what affected their health and come to understand how to remain in good health well into the future.

Crystal messages for good health

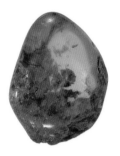

Amber

Be good to yourself. Life is too beautiful for tension and stress. Relax, enjoy and live. Feel the natural vitality within while you simply allow things to happen. Just like you did as a child – do you remember how that felt?

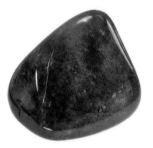

Heliotrope

Be healthy. If you become ill, let go and don't fight it. Allow your inner strength to heal you at your own pace – give yourself space and time to heal. Don't rush it and you will soon discover a new harmony within.

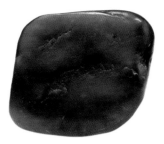

Jade (nephrite)

Get well soon – find the balance between activity and rest. Save your energy, recognise what is doing you good and allow it to do its work. If something annoys you, see if you want to deal with it or if you can simply ignore it. This will help you to relax.

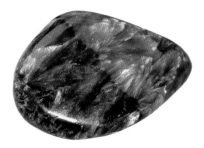

Seraphinite

Keep an eye on yourself. Develop a sense for how you feel or what you might be lacking. Be aware of the first signs of illness and look after yourself. Look on life in general, on yourself and others, with goodwill, and ailments and conflicts will disappear.

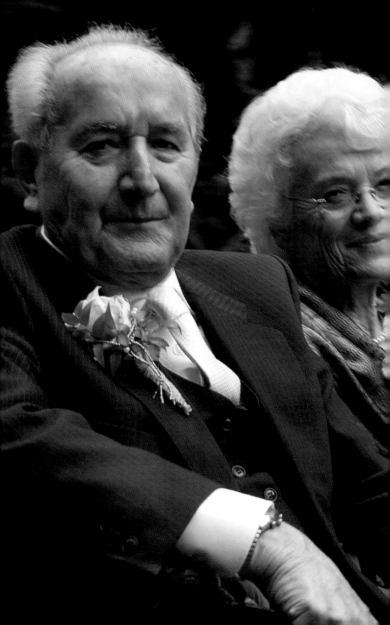

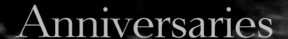

Anniversaries

A day for celebration is here again. It may be a party to celebrate an event we love to remember, or simply to remind ourselves how lucky we are to have enjoyed such happy years. An anniversary doesn't just honour an event, it also recognises all that happened as a result of it and how we have been touched. We are celebrating not just a memory, or the fact that the day has come around again, but we are also remembering the very reason for it.

Crystal messages for anniversaries

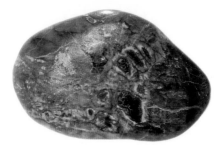

Chrysocolla

If life's highs and lows provide us with valuable experience, if we grow by facing challenges and achieve greater success after failure; if, in hindsight, everything seems to have gone wonderfully well, then we have followed our path beautifully.

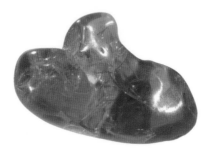

Fire opal

Let us celebrate what was and what is, rather than regretting what might have been. Life is made up of lived experience, what didn't happen never existed. Be happy with life as it is and the future will be full of joy.

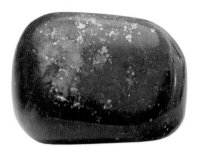

Lapis lazuli

If you follow your own path with dignity and speak the truth when it is important, if you are good and just, helpful and honest – you will find wisdom and be at peace with yourself. If you master life in this way, you will grow in stature yourself.

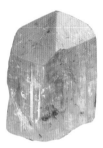

Topaz

What goals have been achieved, what hopes have been realised and what dreams came true? Recognise where your skills and abilities played a part when you answer these questions – and you will see what you have achieved. This is what counts and what endures.

Grief & comfort

Whatever the cause – an accident, suffering, loss or parting from a loved one – grief is an expression of how we honour what has been. It shows that even in our loss we are able to recognise what we had. Grief is therefore a valid and important part of life and comfort is most effective when others similarly respect and honour what has happened. It is only by recognising this, by examining and understanding our loss that we can let go and leave our grief behind.

Crystal messages for giving comfort

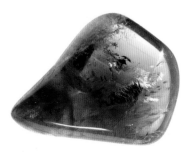

Amethyst

Allow yourself to be sad. Acknowledge what has been lost: closeness, touch, togetherness, understanding. Recognise what you want for yourself and what no longer appears possible. It will hurt, but ultimately this conscious grieving will free you.

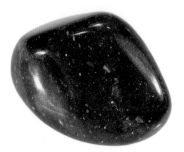

Honduran opal

When everything seems dark, focus upon your hopes. What needs to happen to create a light on the horizon, a small flame in the darkness? Nurture and care for this flame – sometimes miracles do happen...

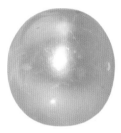

Pearl

Let the tears flow and don't be ashamed of them – they herald relief. Show your pain and you will see that you are still loved. Pain can only subside and die when it is acknowledged and faced.

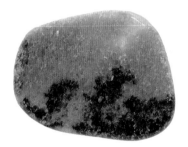

Rhodonite

I feel what you feel. I feel your pain. If you want to unburden yourself, I will always listen to you. If you want me just to be with you in silence, I am there for you. Give yourself time, for even the deepest wounds can heal.

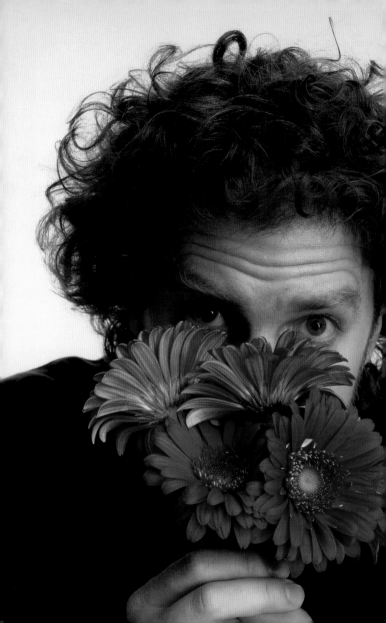

Saying sorry

Misunderstandings, mistakes and hurt feelings are often the result of contact with others; on rare occasions they come about through malicious intent, but they are mostly due to lack of thought and attention. The actual damage caused is generally not as great as the burden of guilt you feel, so asking for forgiveness will free you from that weight and result in happiness all round when granted.

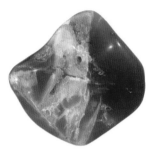

Chrysoprase

You have every right to be annoyed with me, every right to be angry and mad. I didn't act fairly, and what I did was wrong. There is no excuse – I can see that now and I admit it. I would really like to be friends with you again!

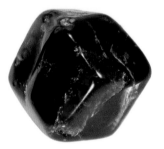

Garnet

I made things difficult for you. I was a burden and often a cause for concern. You received little thanks for all that you did. I recognise that now and ask you to give me another chance; forgive me for what happened. I would like to thank you for your help.

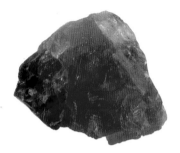

Rhodonite

I know I have hurt you and I ask for your forgiveness; forgiveness for the harsh words, forgiveness for the disregard I showed you, forgiveness for the things I did that I now regret. I cannot undo any of my actions, I can only ask you to forgive me.

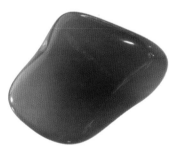

Serpentine

We had an argument and harsh words were said. Instead of making up, we fought over who was right. That hurts me a great deal and I long for peace. Please forgive me for what I did and let us reach out to one another again.

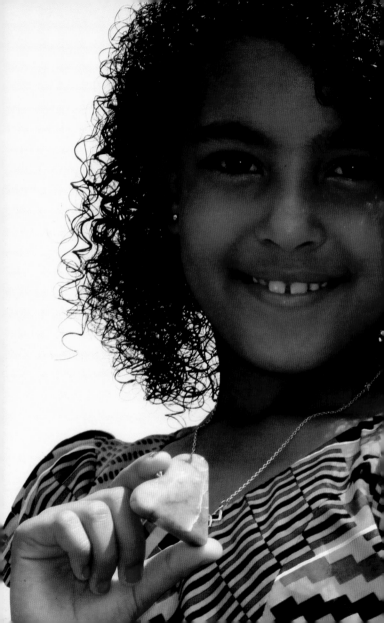

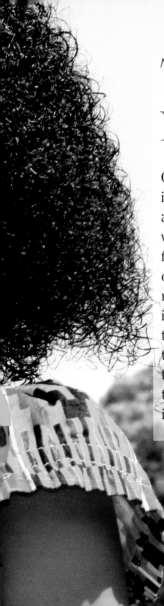

Thank you

Our greatest achievements in life depend upon the help and support of others. Once we realise this fact, we will find that we are rarely lonely or alone. The gratitude that results from this awareness is heartfelt, just as our heart touches another when we say thank you. It is a gift to us and to all those involved, a deep joy that grows deeper the more it is shared...

Crystal messages for giving thanks

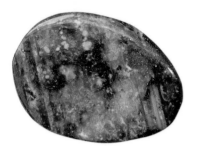

Precious opal

You have made me so happy, thank you for this gift. You have a generous heart and you give with all of it; your eyes light up when others are happy. How beautiful the world would be if everyone were like you!

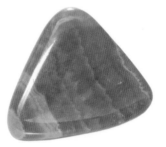

Rhodochrosite

You have touched my heart and I love it every time we meet. We have shared so much joy. I thank you for being you, for the time we spend together, for all the happy moments, and I hope they will continue for a long time to come.

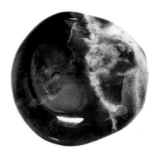

Sardonyx

You were always there when I needed something. You listened when I needed to talk; you had just the right words when I couldn't understand something; your advice prevented me from making mistakes so often. Thank you for being you and for being there for me.

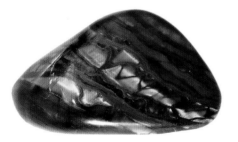

Tiger iron

You were always at my side, ready with help and advice, and your very presence often gave me courage. You believed in my strength and were happy for me when I succeeded, and that in turn gave me strength. I thank you with all my heart!

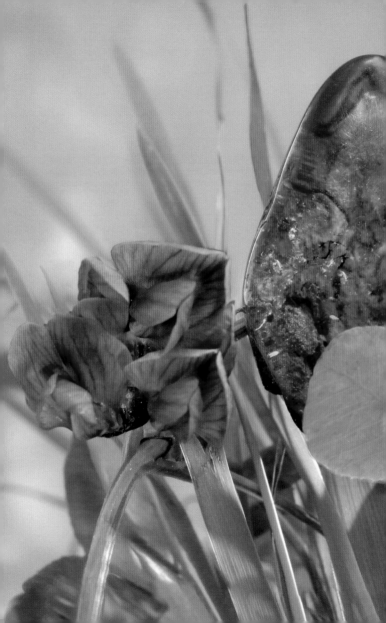

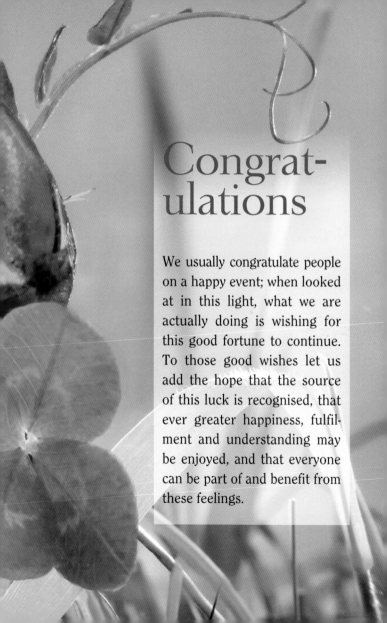

Congrat-
ulations

We usually congratulate people on a happy event; when looked at in this light, what we are actually doing is wishing for this good fortune to continue. To those good wishes let us add the hope that the source of this luck is recognised, that ever greater happiness, fulfilment and understanding may be enjoyed, and that everyone can be part of and benefit from these feelings.

Crystal messages for congratulations

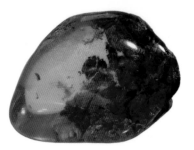

Amber

May you always be happy and joyful and your mind free of worry. Just as you so generously share your gifts with us and with the world, may your every wish come true. Trust in yourself and be sure to stay just the way you are!

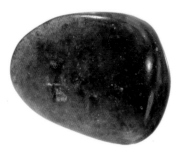

Green aventurine quartz

Recognise what makes you happy and your dreams will come true. Free yourself of the obstacles along your path. Look out for others; this is how you will make friends and travel through life carefree and without impediment.

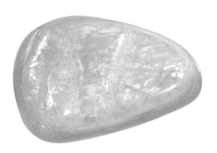

Moonstone

We find fulfilment in what we feel and in those things that touch our senses. Our paths through life will be rich and rewarding if we are guided by an open heart. And for this reason I wish you every happiness.

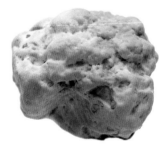

Turquoise

May happiness be with you always. May your eyes always see the right path and your feet take you safely to your destination. May all you do and say help the common good and bring you rich rewards.

Crystals A-Z

Gemstone	Chapter/Topics	Gemstone	Chapter/Topics
Agate	New home, Birth, Pregnancy	Lapis lazuli	Friendship, Exams, Business start-up, Anniversaries
Amber	Birth, Health, Congratulations		
Amethyst	New home, Grief & comfort	Larimar	Career & training
		Malachite	Friendship, Birthdays, Travel
Apophyllite	Career & training		
Aquamarine	Wedding, Business start-up, Travel	Moldavite	Growing up
		Mookaite	New home, Friendship
Azurite	Success	Moonstone	Congratulations
Blue chalcedony	Exams, Starting school	Pearl	Grief & comfort
		Petrified wood	New home
Calcite	Birth		
Carnelian	Nursery	Precious opal	Thank you, Birthdays
Charoite	Work		
Chrysoberyl	Exams	Purpurite	Work
Chrysocolla	Anniversaries, Pregnancy	Pyrite	Starting school
		Rhodo-chrosite	Work, Thank you
Chrysoprase	Saying sorry		
Citrine	Growing up	Rhodonite	Thank you, Grief & comfort
Clear quartz	Growing up	Rose quartz	Birth, Love
Diamond	Wedding	Ruby	Birthdays, Love
Dioptase	Success	Sapphire	Business start-up, Wedding
Dumortierite	Travel, Pregnancy		
Emerald	Wedding	Sardonyx	Thank you
Fire opal	Anniversaries	Seraphinite	Health
Fluorite	Starting school	Serpentine	Saying sorry
Garnet	Saying sorry	Smoky quartz	Work
Gold topaz	Success, Birthdays, Exams		
Green Aven-turine quartz	Congratulations, Nursery	Sodalite	Starting school
		Sugilite	Business start-up
Heliotrope	Health	Sunstone	Pregnancy
Hematite	Nursery	Thulite	Love
Honduran opal	Grief & comfort	Tiger iron	Thank you
		Tiger's eye	Nursery
Jade (nephrite)	Health	Topaz	Career & training, Anniversaries
Jasper	Friendship	Tourmaline	Career & training, Success
Kunzite	Love		
Labradorite	Growing up	Turquoise	Congratulations, Travel

Acknowledgements

I would like to extend my sincere thanks to my publisher, Andreas Lentz, for first suggesting that I write this book, to my wife Anja and my daughter Ariane for their constructive criticism, to Karola Sieber for the beautiful photographs and to Fred Hageneder for the excellent design!

Bibliography

For further inspiration for crystals as gifts or companions and providing support in your life:

M. Gienger, *The Healing Crystal First Aid Manual*, Earthdancer, a Findhorn Press imprint, 2006

M. Gienger, *Die Heilsteine der Hildegard von Bingen*, Neue Erde, 2004

Michael Gienger, *Crystal Power, Crystal Healing*, Cassell Illustrated, 1998

M. Gienger, *Healing Crystals – The A–Z Guide to 555 Gemstones*, Earthdancer, a Findhorn Press imprint, 2014

M. Gienger, *Lexikon der Heilsteine*, Neue Erde, Saarbrücken 2000

Michael Gienger, *Purifying Crystals*, Earthdancer, a Findhorn Press Imprint, 2008

M. Gienger/B. Bruder, *Welcher Heilstein ist das?*, Kosmos, 2009

M. Gienger/J. Goebel, *Edelsteinwasser*, Neue Erde, 2006

M. Gienger/J. Goebel, *Gem Water*, Earthdancer, a Findhorn Press imprint, 2008

The author

Michael Gienger began collecting minerals in 1972 and, from 1985 onwards, immersed himself in the subjects of crystal healing and the energetic qualities of crystals. Michael also gained international acclaim through his research into crystal healing and wrote more than twenty books, some of which have become standard works in their field and have been translated into eleven languages. On 16 November, 2014, following a short illness, Michael Gienger passed away. He has gone but his ideas remain and will not be forgotten.

For further information, see: www.michael-gienger.de, www.steinheilkunde.de, www.fairtrademinerals.de, www.edelstein-massagen.de, www.cairn-elen.de

Consult our catalogue online (with secure order facility) on
www.findhornpress.com
Earthdancer Books is an Imprint of Findhorn Press.
www.earthdancer.co.uk

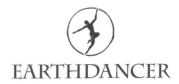

A FINDHORN PRESS IMPRINT